6 ways to unlimited health

Patricia Delacruz

COPYRIGHT

TABLE OF CONTENT

Introduction

Let's face it. Who doesn't want to wake up every morning with unlimited health and vitality to kick off their day with style?

However, it's super hard to perform at peak levels when you always feel tired and sick. Everyone succumbs to the occasional cold or stomach bug, but have you noticed the most successful people seem to be nearly invincible (like they never seem to get tired at all even though they have to manage 50 companies or perform 6 hours on stage)?

It's unbelievable but true. Successful people value themselves highly and invest in their own well-being FIRST. They enjoy life, and don't want illness or injury to disrupt their trajectory. With winter and the holidays ahead, there is no better time to be thinking about staying healthy. To keep you at your best, here are 6 simple habits that will help you stay healthy and enjoy your rise to the top.

1) Eat right

Eating the right foods and the right amounts of foods can help you live a longer, healthier life. Research shows that many illnesses such as diabetes, heart disease, and high blood pressure can be prevented or controlled by simply eating right. Getting the nutrients you need, such as calcium and iron, and keeping your weight under control can help. Try to balance the calories you get from food with the calories you use through physical activity. Remember, it is never too late to start eating right.

Not just that, it is important to not skip breakfast. Research shows that children who skip breakfast generally have poorer nutrition. Their diets contain less:

- Dietary fibre

- Iron

- Calcium

- Vitamins such as riboflavin and niacin.

Skipping breakfast becomes more common as children get older. Some schools have introduced breakfast programs because they were concerned about children who skip breakfast. Study shows that children generally perform better at school when they have breakfast. They are also more likely to maintain a healthy weight when they consume a healthy breakfast.

On the other hand, adults who eat a healthy breakfast are also more likely to be a healthy weight and more productive at work. Breakfast is a way to kickstart your metabolism in the morning (A way to signal your body that it's time to fire up!)

You need to get good nutrition from the calories you need. At all costs, avoid "empty" calories. So what exactly is it?

It basically means food or beverages with calories not made up of basic macronutrients (Healthy Carbohydrates, Proteins and Fats). An excellent example of an empty calories beverage is alcohol. They provide NO nutrients to your body but add on those unwanted calories that make you FAT!

Speaking of fat, also try to avoid food with lots of unhealthy fats or added sugars (or both!). These will seriously make you obese easily if consumed in large quantities.

Secret to lose weight: Opt for FILLING, low-calorie food; rather than sugary, fat-rich CALORIE-DENSE FOOD!

Here's an example: There are 2 foods on the table. One is a piece of carrot cake, and another is a bag of carrots. Both contain the SAME amount of calories.

If you eat a piece of carrot cake, you won't get very much to help your health (and most probably you even crave for MORE!). But let's say you eat the same number of calories in the form of carrots. In that case, you get the calories plus a whole bunch of great nutrients (and you'll feel extremely full).

Keep in mind that most girls should aim to eat no more than 120 or 160 empty calories a day. How can you avoid empty calories? Try cutting back on sugary sodas, fruit drinks, ice cream, cookies, and cake.

Here are some helpful tips of eating healthy

Eat a variety of food, especially:

❖ Vegetables. Choose dark-green leafy and deep-yellow vegetables.

❖ Fruits. Choose berries, melons, citrus fruits or juices.

❖ Whole grains, such as oats, barley, corn, rice, wheat, rice, oats.

❖ Whole grain breads and cereals.

❖ Dry beans (such as soybeans, navy beans and red beans), peanuts, lentils and chickpeas.

❖ Eat food low in fat, saturated fat, and cholesterol, especially:

❖ Fish.

❖ Poultry prepared without skin; lean meat.

❖ Low-fat dairy products.

2) Be physically active

Research shows that physical activity can help prevent at least six diseases: heart disease, high blood pressure, obesity (excess weight), diabetes, osteoporosis, and mental disorders, such as depression. Physical activity also will help you feel better and stay at a healthy weight

Not just that, a number of studies have found that exercise relieves depression. Simply moving your physical body can actually help people out of depression. Physical exercises also block negative thoughts or distract people from daily worries (Some even call it an active form of meditation). Plus, exercising with others provides an opportunity for increased social contact. Increased fitness may lift your mood and even improve sleep patterns.

Research suggests that brisk walking can be just as good for you as an activity such as jogging. A good rule to follow is to do a total of 30 minutes of constant physical activity, such as fast walking, most days of the week.

Before you start being physically active:

1. Talk with your doctor about ways to get started.

2. Choose something that fits into your daily life, such as walking, gardening, raking leaves, or even washing windows.

3. Choose an activity you like, such as dancing or swimming.

4. Try a new activity, like biking.

5. Ask a friend to start with you, or join a group.

Don't quit:

- Make time for physical activity, start slowly, and keep at it.

- If the weather is bad, try an exercise show on TV, watch an exercise tape in your home, walk in the mall, or work around the house.

Physical Activities Guidelines

Here's an excellent guideline to follow:

- Doing any physical activity is better than doing none. If you currently do no physical activity, start by doing some, and gradually build up to the recommended amount.

- Be active on most, preferably all, days every week.

- Accumulate 150 to 300 minutes (2 ½ to 5 hours) of moderate intensity physical activity or 75 to 150 minutes (1 ¼ to 2 ½ hours) of vigorous intensity physical activity, or an equivalent combination of both moderate and vigorous activities, each week.

- Do muscle strengthening activities on at least two days each week.

3) Maintain a positive attitude

Positive thinking is contagious (So is negative). People around you WILL pick your mental moods and are affected accordingly.

Going day-to-day with negative thoughts constantly can weigh a person down both physically and mentally. It is important to shift these negative thoughts into positive ones before it can ruin your day and take a toll on your personal life. Many people do not think to push the thoughts away from our thinking pattern, but we can actually control what thoughts we decide to let affect us.

It is important for us to make time for positivity. It is a given that if you surround yourself and your life with negativity, you will end up in a bad place. Make time in your free time to do things that make you happy personally.

This can be a hobby, reading, sports or exercise. Anything that can be focused on and enjoyed by you is a good distraction from negativity. If you are too focused on aspects of your life that do not promote happiness and positive thinking, those things will end up controlling your life.

When practicing the technique of ignoring negative thoughts, you can also practice introducing positivity in those circumstances. Think of anything positive to replace your negative thoughts. Instead of getting down about something, find something to be happy about and use this optimistic thought to replace your pessimistic thoughts. Practicing this over time, your mind will begin to focus on the good rather than the bad.

Finding a good balance with your emotions is crucial to being a happy and successful person. Take care of your mind, body and soul by making sure negative thoughts do not run your life. Your body will thank you. These personal habits will improve your overall life and therefore your happiness and well-being! Here are 5 tips to overcome negative thoughts.

5 Tips to Overcome Negative Thoughts:

1. Do Yoga Or Meditate

2. Surround yourself with positive people.

3. Remember that no one is perfect and let yourself move forward.

4. Count Your Blessings

5. Don't play the victim. You create your life take responsibility

Hence, always remember to maintain a positive attitude. It has a huge impact on your overall well-being. The Mayo Clinic reports a number of health benefits associated with optimism, including a less depression, reduced risk of death from cardiovascular problems and an increased lifespan.

4) Rely on professionals

There are over 200 types of cancer known, and each type requires its own specialized treatment. Early diagnosis will allow these treatments to begin quickly thereby giving the patient the highest chance for a successful recovery. Nearly 1.5 million people are diagnosed with some form of cancer in the United States, and cancer kills over 500,000 people annually in the United States alone, worldwide that number is closer to 12.5 million cases diagnosed and over 7 million deaths from cancer. Thirty to forty percent of these cases could be prevented and close to one third cured if detected early.

So the question you have to ask yourself is; are you willing to assume you are in good health because you feel fine, or do you think it would be more wise to make an appointment, especially if it has been over a year since you've been, and go get a checkup. What have you got to lose? A few bucks for the visit? Can you put a price on your health? Or even more so, can you put a price on life?

One should get an annual physical check up to make sure everything is as it should be. There is no harm getting regular check ups as it's good for your own body. Do breast or testicular self-exams and get suspicious moles checked out. Getting exams regularly benefits you because if and when something is abnormal, you will get to know about it timely and can consult with your doctor.

Also, it's important for you to play an active role to get the most out of your doctor's visit.

To make the most of your next check-up, here's a quick checklist:

- Review your family health history

- Find out if you are due for any general screenings or vaccinations

- Write down a list of issues and questions to take with you

During your actual doctor's visit, don't be shy about getting your questions answered. Also, if your doctor gives you advice about specific health issues, don't hesitate to take notes. Time is often limited during these exams, but by coming prepared you're sure to get the most out of your checkup.

Regular checkups will provide doctors with a way to spot any health issues early on. Checkups incorporate several tests, including preventative screenings and physical examinations, to check patients' current health and risks. If any problems are found, your doctor will provide information on treatment plans and ways that you can prevent health issues in the future.

Popular health checks include:

- Cervical smear tests (Pap tests) for women

- Blood pressure tests

- Cholesterol level checks

- Body mass index (BMI) and obesity tests

- Diabetes checks

5) Get enough sleep

Sleep loss and sleep disorders are among the most common yet frequently overlooked and readily treatable health problems.
The body requires rest to perform at its best. Not only does short changing sleep take its toll on health, but also relaxation is also required for maximum performance. Successful people schedule time to rest.

Sleeping is as important to your health as eating properly and getting exercise. It is actually damaging to your health to work too hard and not get enough rest. Yet, many people are doing this on a regular basis. In America, we do everything on the go and at a hurried pace. Slowing down and taking a breather is mandatory!

It is estimated 50-70 million US adults have sleep or wakefulness disorder. Notably, snoring is a major indicator of obstructive sleep apnea.

Lack of sleep can affect your overall health and make you prone to serious medical conditions. This includes:

1.Diabetes

2. Obesity

3. High blood pressure

4. Heart disease

How Much Sleep Do We Need? And How Much Sleep Are We Getting?

How much sleep we need varies between individuals but generally changes as we age. The National Institutes of Health suggests that school-age children need at least 10 hours of sleep daily, teens need 9-10 hours, and adults need 7-8 hours. According to data from the National Health Interview Survey, nearly 30% of adults reported an average of ≤6 hours of sleep per day in 2005-2007. In 2009, only 31% of high school students reported getting at least 8 hours of sleep on an average school night.

Sleep Hygiene Tips

- The promotion of good sleep habits and regular sleep is known as sleep hygiene. The following sleep hygiene tips can be used to improve sleep.

- Go to bed at the same time each night and rise at the same time each morning

- Avoid large meals before bedtime

- Avoid nicotine

- Avoid caffeine and alcohol close to bedtime

Here are five ways in which a good night's sleep can boost your health:

1. Sleep boosts mental wellbeing

2. Sleep prevents diabetes

3. Sleep boosts immunity

4. Sleep can slim you

5. Sleep wards off heart disease

6) Take vacation days

Although many Americans receive paid time off through work and 96 percent of people recognize its importance, only 41 percent of workers plan to use all of their vacation days. But taking time off helps us de-stress and that has long-term health implications. Women who only took one vacation every six years or less were nearly eight times more likely to suffer a heart attack or develop heart disease than those who took at least two vacations every year, The New York Times reports.

Everyone needs a vacation once in a while.

Clearly, then, stress is not a good thing. Even people who claim to love the high-pressure lifestyle will admit, in their quieter moments, that there are times when they just want to get away from it all, if only for a short time.

Vacations have the potential to break into the stress cycle. We emerge from a successful vacation feeling ready to take on the world again. We gain perspective on our problems, get to relax with our families and friends, and get a break from our usual routines.

Meeting people from other cultures will teach you that the way you've been looking at the world isn't the way everybody else does. In fact, your point-of-view might have some major blind spots. Seeing the world for yourself will improve your vision and your grip on reality.

Not just that, If you're between jobs, schools, kids, or relationships, traveling around the world can be a perfect way to move from one of these life stages into your next great adventure. A big trip won't just ease your transition into the next stage of your life, it'll give you a chance to reflect on where you've been, where you're going, and where you want to end up.

Seeing the world provides an education that's absolutely impossible to get in school. Travel teaches you economy, politics, history, geography, and sociology in an intense, hands-on way no class will. It makes you feel alive.

We're always told that to seek happiness, you need to try and live in the moment. And it feels almost impossible to do this in the process of your nine-to-five job and in the midst of routine. You've seen it all before, so your mind moves in a habitual motion just passing it all by. But when you travel, your mind is there, you experience so much for the first time that without any effort, and you are present in the moment. It's no wonder so many people become addicted to travelling. It's a constant rush of adrenaline and adventure. The perfect way to reinvigorate yourself, and can be a great way to shake-up your life.